Losing Body Weight in the Weight Room

PREVENT WEIGHT LOSS LEADING TO MUSCLE LOSS. MAINTAINING MUSCLE MASS IS ESSENTIAL TO YOUR HEALTH

Russell Campbell MBA, CSCS

Your Second Opinion, LLC
7735 Willow Cove Circle
Las Vegas, Nevada 89129
campbell@yoursecondopinionllc.com

Book Layout ©2017 BookDesignTemplates.com

Ordering Information:
Quantity sales. Special discounts are available on quantity purchases by corporations, associations, and others. For details, contact the publisher at the address above.

Losing Body Weight in the Weight Room
PREVENT WEIGHT LOSS LEADING TO MUSCLE LOSS. MAINTAINING MUSCLE MASS IS ESSENTIAL TO YOUR HEALTH
ISBN: 9798333504968

Before beginning or adjusting any fitness program, please consult with a licensed health professional who can provide advice based on your personal medical history. This book provides general information to increase awareness, and educate readers. There are differing views on many of the topics covered in this book including benefits, and risk of injury. The publisher assumes no responsibility and expressly disclaims all warranties of any kind, whether expressed or implied to the full extent permitted under applicable laws, relating to your use of this book. Please consult with a health professional if you have any negative side effects.

The author generated some of this text with GPT, OpenAI's large-scale language-generation model. Upon generating draft language, the author reviewed, substantially edited, and revised the language based on his own experience and knowledge and takes ultimate responsibility for the content of this publication.

To Suzy, my Inspiration

Content

Quick Start Guide

"Losing Body Weight in the Weight Room" is about more than just physical transformation. It's about building a healthier, stronger, and more confident you. By combining weight lifting with proper nutrition, recovery, and a positive mindset, you can achieve your weight loss goals while maintaining muscle. This journey is personal, and everyone's path will be different. Stay committed, stay motivated, and enjoy the process. Here's to a healthier, stronger you!

This chapter offers a condensed version of the book's core principles, providing a practical framework for immediate implementation. By following these guidelines, you can start your journey toward losing body weight while maintaining muscle in a structured and effective way.

Understanding Body Composition

Begin by recognizing that body composition is more important than the number on the scale. Focus on reducing body fat while maintaining or increasing lean muscle mass. Lean muscle mass is metabolically active, helping you burn more calories - even at rest.

Nutrition for Weight Loss and Muscle Maintenance

1. **Protein Intake**: Aim for 0.5 grams of protein per pound per day of body weight to support muscle repair and growth.
2. **Carbohydrates**: Focus on complex carbs like whole grains, fruits, and vegetables to fuel your workouts.

3. **Healthy Fats**: Include sources like avocados, nuts, and olive oil to support overall health and hormone production.
4. **Caloric Deficit**: Create a caloric deficit by consuming 500 fewer calories per day than you burn, while limiting the muscle lost from weight loss .

The Science Behind Weight Lifting and Fat Loss

Weight lifting increases your metabolic rate and promotes fat loss through the afterburn effect. It also triggers hormonal responses that enhance muscle growth and fat loss, boosting your resting metabolic rate.

Designing a Weight Lifting Program

1. **Progressive Overload**: Gradually increase the weight, reps, or intensity of your workouts.
2. **Specificity**: Tailor your workouts to your goals, especially focusing on exercises that target major muscle groups.
3. **Periodization**: Vary the intensity (weight) and volume (sets, repetitions) of workouts to optimize performance and recovery.
4. **Compound Movements**: Include squats, deadlifts, bench presses, and rows as the foundation of your routine.

Key Weight Lifting Exercises

Incorporate compound movements (multi-joint) and isolation (single joint) exercises to build a balanced and effective strength training routine. Focus on proper form to prevent injuries and maximize effectiveness.

Cardiovascular Exercise and Weight Lifting

Balance your weight lifting with cardio sessions each week. High-Intensity Interval Training (HIIT) is an advanced training method but it is particularly effective for burning calories and preserving muscle mass.

Recovery and Injury Prevention

1. **Rest**: Ensure adequate sleep and incorporate rest days into your routine.
2. **Stretching**: Include light dynamic stretches before workouts and static stretches afterward.
3. **Mobility Exercises**: Improve flexibility and reduce muscle stiffness to prevent injuries.

Maintaining a Positive Mindset

Set achievable goals and celebrate progress. Understand that setbacks are part of the journey. And there is no such thing as a bad workout! Every effort helps in the long run.

Stay motivated by tracking your progress, joining a fitness community, or finding a workout buddy. Exercise not only improves physical health but also mental well-being, reducing stress and enhancing mood.

Consider working with a trainer or coach at least at the beginning to become comfortable and competent with weight training.

Tracking Progress

Keep a workout journal to record exercises, weights, reps, and your feelings after each session. Regularly measure body composition, strength gains, and overall fitness. Adjust your diet and workout plan based on your progress, and change your routine or increase intensity if you hit a plateau.

Quick Start Checklist
1. **Nutrition: Calculate your protein, carb, and fat needs. Plan meals around these macronutrients.**
2. **Exercise: Design a weight lifting program with compound movements and add cardio sessions.**
3. **Recovery: Prioritize sleep, rest days, and stretching.**
4. **Mindset: Set realistic goals, track progress, and stay positive**

Who Am I

I'm just like you, I have a few extra pounds on me, But this hasn't stopped me from enjoying life. I know that working out makes me feel great and enables me to be as active as I want to be.

You know what's even cooler? I enjoy coaching others who have discovered the magic of the weight room in achieving fitness and weight loss goals.

Not only do I have the hands-on experience, but I've also got the education to back it up. I'm a Certified Strength & Conditioning Specialist, and a USA Weightlifting Certified Coach. So, I've got the know-how to help you reach your fitness goals by staying active and healthy.

Also, I keep up-to-date with all the latest scientific research. I'm always learning and growing, so my training programs are based on the latest evidence.

All of this knowledge and experience go into my coaching efforts for people like you. I love working with people of all ages, and it's a true passion of mine to help you improve your physical capacity and stay healthy for life!

So, if you're ready, I'm here to show you the ropes and take your physical health to the next level, injury-free. Together, we'll work hard, have fun, and make you the best that you can be! Let's do this!

Understanding Body Composition

Body composition is a more precise indicator of health than body weight alone. It distinguishes between the weight of fat and lean tissue, providing a clearer picture of your fitness level. Lean muscle mass is particularly important because it influences your metabolic rate. Muscle tissue requires more energy to maintain than fat tissue, meaning that people with higher muscle mass burn more calories at rest. This is why strength training is often recommended for weight loss and management.

The body consists of various components: water, protein, minerals, and fat. The proportion of these components varies among individuals and can change over time due to factors such as diet, exercise, and aging. For example, the water content can fluctuate with hydration levels, while muscle and fat proportions can be altered through exercise and diet.

The Role of Lean Muscle Mass

Lean muscle mass is not just about aesthetics; it's about functionality and health. Muscles are involved in nearly every movement and activity, from walking and lifting objects to maintaining posture and balance. As we age, maintaining muscle mass becomes even more critical. Sarcopenia, or the loss of muscle mass due to aging, can lead to decreased mobility, higher risk of falls, and overall decline in physical function.

Strength training helps combat sarcopenia by stimulating muscle growth and improving muscle strength. This type of exercise involves working against resistance to enhance the strength and size of your muscles. By incorporating strength training into your routine, you can preserve and even increase your muscle mass, which supports better metabolism and overall health.

Setting Realistic Goals

When it comes to body composition, setting realistic and attainable goals is essential. Rather than aiming for rapid weight loss, focus on gradual and sustainable changes. Aiming to lose about 1 pound of fat per week is a reasonable goal. And you want to lose fat, not muscle, which is crucial for long-term health.

In addition to fat loss, it's important to set goals for maintaining or increasing muscle mass. This can be achieved by incorporating regular strength training exercises into your fitness routine. Aim for at least two to three sessions per week, focusing on all major muscle groups.

Measuring Body Composition

There are several methods to measure body composition, ranging from simple to sophisticated. One of the most common methods is the Body Mass Index (BMI), which uses height and weight to estimate body fat. However, BMI does not differentiate between muscle and fat, so it may not be the most accurate indicator for everyone.

More precise methods include:

- **Skinfold measurements**: Using calipers to measure the thickness of skinfolds at various body sites.
- **Bioelectrical impedance analysis (BIA)**: Using a small electrical current to estimate body composition based on the resistance of body tissues.
- **Dual-energy X-ray absorptiometry (DEXA)**: A detailed scan that measures bone density and body composition.
- **Hydrostatic weighing**: Measuring body density by comparing weight on land and in water.

Conclusion

Understanding and improving your body composition is key to achieving long-term health and fitness goals. By focusing on preserving and building lean muscle mass through strength training, you can enhance your metabolic rate, improve your physical function, and achieve a healthier body. Set realistic goals, measure your progress, and stay committed to your fitness journey. With dedication and the right approach, you can transform your body and your health.

Nutrition for Weight Loss and Muscle Maintenance

Nutrition plays a pivotal role in weight loss and muscle maintenance. The three macronutrients—proteins, carbohydrates, and fats—each have a unique role. Protein is crucial for muscle repair and growth. Aim for at least 0.5 grams of protein per pound per day of body weight. Carbohydrates are your body's primary energy source, especially for high-intensity workouts. Focus on complex carbs like whole grains, fruits, and vegetables. Healthy fats, found in avocados, nuts, and olive oil as examples, support hormone production and overall health.

Creating a caloric deficit, where you consume fewer calories than you burn, is essential for weight loss. However, it's vital to do this without sacrificing muscle. Losing one pound per week is a reasonable goal. Eating 500 calories a day less will help to achieve that goal and preserve muscle.

Distribute your meals evenly throughout the day, including protein in each meal, to keep your metabolism steady and support muscle maintenance. Hydration is also key. Drink plenty of water to support your workouts and recovery.

The Role of Macronutrients

Proteins: Protein is crucial for muscle repair and growth. It provides the building blocks (amino acids) necessary for muscle tissue synthesis. For individuals aiming to lose weight while maintaining muscle mass, it's important to consume adequate protein. Aim for at least 0.5 grams of protein per pound per day of body weight. High-quality protein sources include lean meats, poultry, fish, eggs, dairy products, legumes, and plant-based proteins. Consuming protein throughout the day, especially before and after workouts, helps maximize muscle protein synthesis.

Carbohydrates: Carbohydrates are the body's primary energy source, particularly for high-intensity workouts and strength training. They fuel your muscles and brain, providing the necessary energy to perform and recover from exercise. Focus on consuming complex carbohydrates, such as whole grains, fruits, and vegetables. These sources provide a steady release of energy and are rich in essential nutrients and fiber, which aids in digestion and not feeling hungry. Avoid simple sugars and refined carbs, which can lead to spikes and crashes in blood sugar levels.

Fats: Healthy fats are essential for hormone production, brain function, and overall health. They also provide a concentrated source of energy. Incorporate healthy fats found in avocados, nuts, seeds, olive oil, and fatty fish into your diet. These fats support cell structure and function, and help with the absorption of fat-soluble vitamins (A, D, E, and K). Avoid trans fats and limit saturated fats, which can negatively impact cardiovascular health.

Creating a Caloric Deficit

A caloric deficit, where you consume fewer calories than you burn, is essential for weight loss. However, it's important to achieve this deficit without sacrificing muscle mass. Drastic calorie cuts can lead to muscle loss and a decrease in metabolic rate. A slower metabolic rate undermines your ability to lose weight.

Instead, aim for a moderate calorie reduction that supports steady, sustainable weight loss. Typically, a deficit of 500 calories per day is recommended, which can lead to a weight loss of about 1 pound per week.

Distribute your meals evenly throughout the day, including a source of protein in each meal, to keep your metabolism steady and support muscle maintenance. Frequent, balanced meals help maintain energy levels, prevent overeating, and support muscle repair and growth.

Importance of Hydration

Hydration is also key. Drinking plenty of water is crucial for overall health and particularly important during weight loss and exercise. Water aids in digestion, nutrient absorption, and temperature regulation. It also helps transport nutrients to your muscles and remove waste products. Aim to drink at least 8-10 cups of water per day, more if you're engaging in intense physical activity. If you are working out for more than one hour at a time, you'll need to add carbs and electrolytes to your water.

Proper hydration can improve workout performance, reduce the risk of injury, and aid in recovery. Losing water weight alone will undermine your workout performance and is not healthy.

Practical Tips for Nutritional Success

- **Meal Planning**: Plan your meals ahead of time to ensure a balanced intake of nutrients. This can help you avoid unhealthy choices and control portion sizes.
- **Mindful Eating**: Pay attention to your hunger and fullness cues. Eat slowly and savor your meals to enhance satisfaction and prevent over-eating.
- **Snacking**: Choose healthy snacks that combine protein, healthy fats, and complex carbohydrates. Examples include Greek yogurt with berries, apple slices with almond butter, or a handful of nuts.
- **Supplements**: While whole foods should be your primary nutrient source, supplements like whey protein or multivitamins can help fill nutritional gaps, especially when dietary restrictions are in place.
-

Conclusion

By understanding and implementing these nutritional strategies, you can effectively lose weight while maintaining muscle mass. A balanced diet that emphasizes adequate protein, complex carbohydrates, healthy fats, and proper hydration will support your weight loss goals and enhance your overall health.

Remember, consistency is key. Making small, sustainable changes to your eating habits will lead to long-term success.

!

The Science Behind Weight Lifting and Fat Loss

Weight lifting, or resistance training, is incredibly effective for fat loss and muscle maintenance. Weight lifting increases your metabolic rate, leading to calorie burn even after your workout. This is known as the afterburn effect or Excess Post-exercise Oxygen Consumption (EPOC).

Lifting weights also triggers hormonal responses that promote muscle growth and fat loss. Testosterone and growth hormone levels increase, aiding in muscle repair and growth. The more muscle you have, the higher your resting metabolic rate, which means you burn more calories at rest. This makes weight lifting a powerful tool for transforming your body composition.

The Afterburn Effect

EPOC refers to the increased rate of oxygen intake following strenuous activity. After an intense weight lifting session, your body continues to consume oxygen at a higher rate to repair muscles, replenish energy stores, and restore your body to its resting state. This process requires energy, which means you continue to burn calories even when you are not actively exercising. Studies have shown that EPOC can last for up to 24-48 hours post-exercise, significantly boosting your overall calorie expenditure.

Hormonal Responses

Lifting weights triggers hormonal responses that promote muscle growth and fat loss. Two key hormones involved are testosterone and growth hormone.

Testosterone is crucial for muscle repair and growth. It enhances protein synthesis, which is the process by which your body builds new muscle tissue. Growth hormone, on the other hand, stimulates fat metabolism and helps in muscle recovery and growth. These hormonal boosts are essential for anyone looking to lose fat while preserving or building muscle mass.

Metabolic Rate and Muscle Mass

The more muscle you have, the higher your resting metabolic rate (RMR). Muscle tissue is metabolically active, meaning it requires more energy to maintain than fat tissue. For every pound of muscle gained, your body burns an additional 6-10 calories per day at rest. This may not sound like much, but it adds up over time and can significantly impact your overall calorie expenditure.

By increasing your muscle mass through weight lifting, you enhance your body's ability to burn calories, even when you are not working out. This makes weight lifting a powerful tool for transforming your body composition, as it helps to create a calorie deficit necessary for fat loss while preserving lean muscle mass.

Practical Application

To maximize the benefits of weight lifting for fat loss, it's important to incorporate compound exercises that engage multiple muscle groups. Exercises such as squats, deadlifts, bench presses, and rows are highly effective because they require a significant amount of energy and stimulate the release of muscle-building hormones. Additionally, incorporating progressive overload—gradually increasing the weight or resistance in your workouts—ensures continuous muscle growth and adaptation.

Another effective strategy is to include high-intensity interval training (HIIT) with your weight lifting regimen. HIIT involves short bursts of intense exercise followed by brief periods of rest or lower-intensity exercise. This not only enhances EPOC but also improves cardiovascular fitness and promotes greater fat loss. Keep in mind that HIIT is considered advanced training. Beginners should work their way up to it.

Nutrition and Recovery

Proper nutrition and recovery are vital components of a successful weight lifting program.. Ensuring you get enough sleep and allowing time for muscle recovery are equally important. Lastly, Overtraining can lead to injuries and impede progress, so it's crucial to listen to your body and incorporate rest days into your routine.

Conclusion

Weight lifting offers a scientifically-backed approach to fat loss and muscle maintenance. By understanding the afterburn effect, hormonal responses, and the role of muscle mass in metabolism, you can effectively use weight lifting to achieve your weight loss goals. Incorporate compound exercises, practice progressive overload, and pair your workouts with proper nutrition and recovery strategies to transform your body composition and improve your overall health

Designing a Weight Lifting Program

A well-designed weight lifting program is crucial for effective weight loss and muscle maintenance. The key principles are progressive overload, specificity, and periodization. Progressive overload means gradually increasing the weight, reps, or intensity of your workouts to continually challenge your muscles. Specificity involves tailoring your workouts to your specific goals, while focusing on exercises that target major muscle groups.

Periodization is the systematic planning of training cycles. It involves varying the intensity and volume of workouts to optimize performance and recovery. A balanced program includes compound movements (like squats and deadlifts), which work multiple muscle groups, and isolation exercises (like bicep curls), which target specific muscles. Structure your weekly workouts to include two to three weight lifting sessions, ensuring you allow adequate rest and recovery time between sessions.

Progressive Overload

Progressive overload is the cornerstone of any effective strength training program. It involves gradually increasing the weight, repetitions, or intensity of your workouts to continually challenge your muscles. Without progressive overload, your muscles will adapt to the workload, and you will hit a plateau. To avoid this, you can:

- **Increase Weight**: Gradually add more weight to your exercises as your strength improves. Even small increments on a regular basis can make a big difference over time.

- **Increase Repetitions**: If you can't add weight, try increasing the number of repetitions. This also challenges your muscles and promotes growth. However, generally keep the number of repetitions below 10 to maintain the focus on strength.
- **Increase Intensity**: Shorten rest periods between sets or add intensity techniques like supersets or drop sets to keep your muscles under constant tension.

Specificity

Specificity means tailoring your workouts to your specific goals. For weight loss and muscle maintenance, focus on exercises that target major muscle groups. Compound movements, which involve multiple joints and muscles, are particularly effective. These include:

- **Squats**: Work the quads, hamstrings, glutes, and core.
- **Deadlifts**: Engage the entire posterior chain, including the hamstrings, glutes, lower back, and traps.
- **Bench Press**: Targets the chest, shoulders, and triceps.
- **Rows**: Strengthen the back, biceps, and core.

In addition to compound movements, include isolation exercises to target specific muscles and address any imbalances. For example:

- **Bicep Curls**: Focus on the biceps.
- **Tricep Extensions**: Target the triceps.

Periodization

Periodization is the systematic planning of training cycles to optimize performance and recovery. This involves varying the intensity and volume of your workouts over different periods. A well-structured periodization plan can prevent overtraining, reduce the risk of injury, and promote continuous progress. Typical phases include:

- **Preparation Phase**: Focus on building a solid foundation with lower intensity (less weight) and higher volume (more reps) workouts. This phase lasts about 4-6 weeks.
- **Hypertrophy Phase**: Increase the intensity and volume to build muscle size. This phase typically lasts 4-8 weeks.
- **Strength Phase**: Focus on lifting heavier weights with lower repetitions (6 or less) to focus on building strength. This phase can last 3-6 weeks.
- **Deload Phase**: Reduce the intensity and volume to allow your body to recover. This phase usually lasts 1-2 weeks.
-

Structuring Your Weekly Workouts

To ensure balanced development and adequate recovery, structure your weekly workouts to include two to three weight lifting sessions. Here's a sample weekly plan:
- **Day 1**: Lower Body (Squats, Deadlifts, Lunges)
- **Day 2**: Rest or Active Recovery
- **Day 3**: Upper Body (Bench Press, Rows, Shoulder Press)
- **Day 4**: Rest or Active Recovery
- **Day 5**: Full Body (Compound Movements)

Rest and Recovery

Adequate rest and recovery are essential components of a successful weight lifting program. Muscles grow and repair during rest periods, not while you are working out. Ensure you get at least three days of rest from weight training each week and focus on getting quality sleep, which is crucial for muscle recovery and overall health.

!

Key Weight Lifting Exercises

Certain exercises are particularly effective for fat loss and muscle maintenance. Compound movements are the cornerstone of any weight lifting program. Squats, deadlifts, bench presses, and rows engage multiple muscle groups, burn more calories, and stimulate muscle growth. These exercises should form the foundation of your routine.

Isolation exercises, such as bicep curls and tricep extensions, can be added to target specific muscles and create balanced development.

Focus on proper form and technique to prevent injuries and maximize effectiveness. Incorporate a mix of both types of exercises to ensure a comprehensive approach to strength training.

Compound Movements

Squats Squats are one of the most fundamental exercises for building strength and burning fat. They engage the quadriceps, hamstrings, glutes, lower back, and core. The squat is often referred to as the "king of exercises" because of its ability to activate large muscle groups, leading to significant calorie burn and muscle growth. Proper form is crucial to prevent injuries; ensure your knees track straight over your toes, your back stays straight, and you go as deep as your flexibility allows. Variations like front squats and goblet squats can also be included to target muscles differently and add variety to your routine.

Deadlifts Deadlifts are another essential compound movement that targets the posterior chain, including the hamstrings, glutes, lower back, traps, and forearms. This exercise is highly effective for increasing overall strength and boosting metabolic rate. When performing deadlifts, maintain a neutral spine, keep the bar close to your body, and lift with your legs, not your back. Variations such as sumo deadlifts and Romanian deadlifts can be incorporated to emphasize different muscle groups and prevent workout monotony.

Bench Press The bench press primarily works the chest, shoulders, and triceps. It is a staple in any strength training program and is excellent for building upper body muscle mass. To perform a bench press, lie on a bench, grasp the barbell with a shoulder-width grip, and lower it to your chest before pressing it back up. Control the weight and avoid bouncing the bar off your chest. Incline and decline bench presses can be added to target the upper and lower parts of the chest respectively. Standing presses are another alternative.

Rows Rows, such as barbell rows or dumbbell rows, target the muscles of the upper back, including the lats, traps, and rhomboids, as well as the biceps and forearms. These exercises are crucial for developing a balanced physique and improving posture. Focus on pulling with your back muscles rather than your arms and keeping your movements controlled. Bent-over rows and single-arm dumbbell rows are effective variations to include in your program.

Isolation Exercises

While compound movements should form the foundation of your routine, isolation exercises can be added to target specific muscles and create balanced development. These exercises are particularly useful for addressing muscle imbalances and enhancing muscle definition.

Bicep Curls Bicep curls are effective for targeting the biceps, enhancing arm strength, and improving muscle tone. Perform curls with dumbbells, a barbell, or an EZ-curl bar, ensuring you maintain strict form to maximize effectiveness and prevent injury. Variations such as hammer curls and concentration curls can help target different parts of the biceps.

Tricep Extensions Tricep extensions are essential for developing the triceps, which make up a significant portion of the upper arm. Perform them with dumbbells, a barbell, or a cable machine. Overhead tricep extensions and tricep kickbacks are effective variations to include.

Lateral Raises Lateral raises target the shoulder muscles, particularly the deltoids, and are crucial for building a well-rounded upper body. Perform them with light dumbbells or a cable machine, ensuring you lift with your shoulders and not your traps. Incorporate front raises and reverse flyes to target different parts of the shoulder.

Leg Press The leg press is a compound movement that complements squats and deadlifts, focusing on the quadriceps, hamstrings, and glutes. Adjust the foot placement on the platform to target different parts of the legs and add variety to your routine.

Lat Pulldowns Lat pulldowns target the latissimus dorsi and are excellent for building a strong back. Use a cable machine, pulling the bar down to your chest while maintaining an upright posture. Variations like close-grip pulldowns and single-arm pulldowns can help target different areas of the back.

By incorporating a mix of compound and isolation exercises, you can create a balanced and effective weight lifting program. Focus on proper form and technique to prevent injuries and maximize the effectiveness of each exercise. This comprehensive approach to strength training will ensure you achieve your weight loss and muscle maintenance goals.

Cardiovascular Exercise & Weight Lifting

While weight lifting is crucial for muscle maintenance, cardiovascular exercise also plays a role in a balanced fitness program. Cardio helps burn additional calories, improving cardiovascular health and aiding in weight loss.

High-Intensity Interval Training (HIIT) is a particularly effective advanced exercise. It involves short bursts of intense exercise followed by rest periods, maximizing calorie burn and preserving muscle.

Balancing cardio with weight lifting can be challenging. Aim to incorporate two to three cardio sessions per week, focusing on HIIT or moderate-intensity activities like brisk walking or cycling. Ensure your cardio sessions do not interfere with your recovery from weight lifting by doing cardio on non-weight training days or by doing cardio at the end of your weight training workouts.. The goal is to create a complementary relationship between the two, optimizing fat loss while maintaining muscle.

The Role of Cardiovascular Exercise

Cardio exercises, such as running, cycling, swimming, and even brisk walking, elevate your heart rate, improve lung capacity, and enhance overall endurance. Regular cardio can reduce the risk of chronic diseases such as heart disease, diabetes, and hypertension. It also plays a vital role in calorie expenditure, which is essential for weight loss.

High-Intensity Interval Training (HIIT)

High-Intensity Interval Training (HIIT) is particularly effective for those looking to maximize calorie burn and preserve muscle. HIIT involves short bursts of intense exercise followed by rest periods or low-intensity exercise.

This type of training keeps your heart rate elevated, promoting higher calorie burn both during and after the workout due to the Excess Post-exercise Oxygen Consumption (EPOC) effect. HIIT can be applied to various forms of exercise, including running, cycling, or even bodyweight exercises.

For example, a typical HIIT session might include 30 seconds of sprinting followed by 1 minute of walking, repeated for 20-30 minutes. This approach not only helps in burning fat but also saves time compared to traditional steady-state cardio.

Balancing Cardio with Weight Lifting

Balancing cardio with weight lifting can be challenging but is essential for a well-rounded fitness program. Here are some strategies to integrate cardio into your routine without compromising your weight lifting goals:

1. **Separate Cardio and Weight Lifting Sessions**: If possible, perform your cardio and weight lifting on different days or at different times of the day. This approach allows you to fully focus on each type of workout and ensures that cardio does not interfere with your recovery from weight lifting.

2. **Post-Weight Lifting Cardio**: If you prefer to do both in the same session, perform weight lifting first, followed by cardio. This sequence ensures that your energy and strength are maximized for lifting weights, which is crucial for muscle maintenance and growth.

3. **Moderate-Intensity Cardio**: Incorporate moderate-intensity cardio exercises like brisk walking, cycling, or swimming on your non-lifting days. These activities help in burning additional calories without overly taxing your muscles and impairing recovery from weight training.

4. **HIIT**: As mentioned earlier, HIIT is an excellent choice for cardio because it is time-efficient and effective for fat loss. Incorporate HIIT sessions two to three times per week. For example, a 20-minute HIIT workout can provide significant benefits and complement your weight lifting routine.

Optimizing Fat Loss and Muscle Maintenance

The goal is to create a complementary relationship between cardio and weight lifting.

By incorporating both cardiovascular exercise and weight lifting into your fitness routine, you can achieve a balanced approach to weight loss and muscle maintenance. This comprehensive strategy will help you reach your fitness goals more effectively and sustainably.

Recovery and Injury Prevention

Recovery is as important as the workouts themselves. Muscles grow and repair during rest, not during exercise. Ensure you get adequate sleep, as it's crucial for muscle recovery and overall health. Incorporate rest days into your weekly routine to allow your muscles to heal and grow stronger.

Stretching and mobility exercises should be part of your routine to improve flexibility, reduce muscle stiffness, and prevent injuries. Dynamic stretches before workouts and static stretches afterward can enhance your performance and recovery.

Lastly, if you experience any pain or discomfort, don't ignore it. Address injuries promptly and consult a professional if needed.

Importance of Sleep

Sleep is crucial for muscle recovery and overall well-being. During deep sleep, the body releases growth hormones that facilitate muscle repair and growth. Aim for at least 7 hours of quality sleep per night. Poor sleep can hinder your progress, leading to increased fatigue, reduced muscle recovery, and impaired cognitive function. Establish a consistent sleep schedule, create a restful environment, and avoid stimulants like caffeine before bedtime to improve sleep quality.

Incorporating Rest Days

Rest days are essential to allow your muscles to heal and grow stronger. Overtraining can lead to fatigue, decreased performance, and increased risk of injury. Incorporate at least one or two rest days into your weekly routine. These rest days can include light activities like walking or yoga, but avoid intense workouts to give your body the time it needs to recover.

Stretching and Mobility Exercises

Stretching and mobility exercises should be an integral part of your routine to improve flexibility, reduce muscle stiffness, and prevent injuries. Dynamic stretches before workouts prepare your muscles for the exercise ahead by increasing blood flow and enhancing range of motion. Examples of dynamic stretching include leg swings, arm circles, and torso twists. Static stretches after workouts help in relaxing and lengthening the muscles, promoting recovery and reducing soreness. Hold each stretch for at least 30 seconds, focusing on major muscle groups.

Hydration and Nutrition

Proper hydration is vital for muscle recovery. Water helps transport nutrients to your muscles and removes waste products. Aim to drink at least 8-10 glasses of water daily, and increase intake on workout days. Additionally, electrolytes lost through sweat need to be replenished especially during longer workouts. Include foods rich in potassium, magnesium, and sodium, or consider an electrolyte supplement.

Nutrition also plays a key role in recovery. Consuming a balanced diet with adequate protein, carbohydrates, and fats supports muscle repair and replenishes energy stores.

Active Recovery

Active recovery involves low-intensity activities that promote blood flow to the muscles without causing further strain. Activities like light jogging, swimming, or yoga can help reduce muscle stiffness and speed up recovery. Active recovery can be incorporated on rest days or after intense workout sessions.

Listening to Your Body

Pay attention to your body's signals. If you experience pain or discomfort, do not ignore it. Pain can be an indication of overtraining, improper form, or an injury. Address any issues promptly to prevent them from worsening. Ice packs, compression, and elevation can help manage acute injuries. For persistent or severe pain, consult a healthcare professional or physical therapist.

Professional Support

Consider seeking professional support for personalized recovery strategies. A physical therapist, massage therapist, or sports physician can provide tailored advice and treatment to enhance recovery and prevent injuries. Regular check-ups and assessments can help identify potential issues before they become serious problems.

Recovery Tools

Utilize recovery tools such as foam rollers, massage guns, and compression garments to aid in muscle recovery. Foam rolling can release muscle tension and improve blood flow. Massage guns provide deep tissue massage, helping to alleviate soreness and tightness. Compression garments can reduce muscle swelling and promote faster recovery.

In conclusion, prioritizing recovery and injury prevention is crucial for achieving long-term success in your fitness journey. By incorporating proper sleep, rest days, stretching, hydration, nutrition, active recovery, and listening to your body, you can enhance your performance, maintain muscle, and reduce the risk of injuries. Remember, the journey to fitness is a marathon, not a sprint. Take care of your body, and it will take care of you.

A positive mindset is key to any successful fitness journey. Set achievable goals and celebrate your progress along the way. Understand that setbacks are part of the process. Stay motivated by tracking your progress, joining a fitness community, or finding a workout buddy.

Mental Health and Motivation

Exercise has profound mental health benefits. It reduces stress, anxiety, and depression, and improves mood and overall well-being. The social aspect of working out, whether in a gym or with friends, can provide additional motivation and a sense of community. Stay focused on your goals, but also enjoy the journey and the improvements you see in yourself.

A positive mindset is the cornerstone of any successful fitness journey. It's the driving force that keeps you motivated, focused, and resilient, especially when the going gets tough. Developing a positive outlook can transform your approach to fitness, making the process more enjoyable and sustainable. Here's how to cultivate a positive mindset and harness it for long-term success.

Setting Achievable Goals

Setting realistic, achievable goals is essential. Start by defining clear, specific objectives that you can measure. Instead of saying, "I want to lose weight," set a target like, "I aim to lose 10 pounds in three months by exercising three times a week and eating a balanced diet." Break down these larger goals into smaller milestones. Each milestone you achieve provides a sense of accomplishment and motivates you to keep pushing forward.

Celebrating small victories is equally important. Every pound lost, every inch shed, and every new weight lifted is a step closer to your ultimate goal. Recognize and reward yourself for these achievements. This could be as simple as a verbal acknowledgment, treating yourself to a new workout outfit, or enjoying a healthy snack. Celebrating progress reinforces your commitment and helps maintain enthusiasm.

Embracing Setbacks

Understand that setbacks are a natural part of any fitness journey. There will be days when you miss a workout, indulge in unhealthy food, or feel de-motivated. Instead of being harsh on yourself, view these setbacks as learning opportunities. Reflect on what led to the setback and how you can prevent it in the future. This approach fosters resilience and a growth mindset, crucial for long-term success.

Staying Motivated

Tracking your progress is a powerful motivator. Keep a fitness journal or use a mobile app to log your workouts, dietary intake, and any changes in your body measurements. Visualizing your progress can be incredibly satisfying and provides tangible proof of your hard work. It also helps identify patterns and areas that need improvement.

Joining a fitness community or finding a workout buddy can significantly enhance your motivation. Being part of a group with similar goals creates a support system where you can share experiences, challenges, and successes. Group activities and shared workouts make exercise more enjoyable and less of a solitary task. The camaraderie and accountability within a fitness community can push you to stay committed, even when your motivation wanes.

Enjoying the Journey

While staying focused on your goals is important, it's equally crucial to enjoy the journey. Find joy in the improvements you see in yourself, both physically and mentally. Appreciate the increased energy levels, the better mood, and the growing strength. Celebrate the fact that you are taking active steps towards a healthier, happier you.

Practical Tips for Cultivating a Positive Mindset
1. Daily Affirmations: Start your day with positive affirmations. Remind yourself of your goals and the progress you've made.

2. Visualization: Visualize your success. Picture yourself achieving your fitness goals and how great it will feel.
3. Mindfulness: Practice mindfulness and stay present during your workouts. Focus on your movements, breathing, and the sensations in your body.
4. Positive Environment: Surround yourself with positivity. Follow motivational social media accounts, read inspiring stories, and engage with positive people.
5. Gratitude: Keep a gratitude journal. Write down things you are thankful for, including your health and the ability to exercise.

In conclusion, cultivating a positive mindset is key to any successful fitness journey. By setting achievable goals, celebrating progress, embracing setbacks, staying motivated, and enjoying the process, you can transform your approach to fitness. Remember, a positive outlook not only enhances your physical health but also your mental well-being. Stay focused, stay positive, and enjoy the journey to a healthier you

Tracking Progress

Tracking your progress helps you stay motivated and make necessary adjustments. Measure your body composition, strength gains, and overall fitness regularly. Keep a workout journal to record your exercises, weights, reps, and how you feel after each session.

Adjust your diet and workout plan based on your progress. If you hit a plateau, consider changing your routine or increasing the intensity of your workouts. Long-term maintenance involves continuing the habits you've developed, staying active, and making healthy food choices.

Tracking your progress is a cornerstone of any successful fitness journey, especially when it comes to losing weight and maintaining muscle. It keeps you motivated, provides tangible evidence of your efforts, and helps you make necessary adjustments to your workout and diet plans. Here's how you can effectively track your progress and ensure you're on the right path to achieving your fitness goals.

The Importance of Measuring Progress

Regularly measuring your body composition, strength gains, and overall fitness levels is crucial. Body composition measurements help you understand the changes in your fat and lean mass. Use tools like body fat calipers, bioelectrical impedance scales, or even DEXA scans if available, to get accurate readings. These measurements can show you whether you're losing fat and maintaining or even gaining muscle, which is more meaningful than just watching the scale.

Strength gains are another critical metric. Track how much weight you lift, how many reps and sets you perform, and how your strength improves over time. Noticing improvements in your strength can be incredibly motivating and is a clear indicator that your fitness program is working.

If you are new to weigh training or have not lifted weights in a long time, you may be very surprised by how quickly you make significant progress.

Keeping a Workout Journal

A workout journal is an invaluable tool. Record each exercise, the weights you used, the number of reps and sets, and how you felt during and after the session. This not only helps you keep track of what you've accomplished but also allows you to identify patterns and make adjustments as needed. For example, if you notice you're consistently lifting heavier weights or completing more reps, it's a sign of progress.

Additionally, document your daily nutrition intake. Note what you eat, the portion sizes, and the macronutrient breakdown. This can help you identify any dietary adjustments needed to support your fitness goals. Tracking your food intake alongside your workouts provides a comprehensive picture of your progress and helps you stay accountable.

Adjusting Your Plan

Hitting a plateau can be frustrating, but it's a natural part of the fitness journey. If your progress stalls, it might be time to adjust your workout routine or diet. Consider incorporating different types of exercises, increasing the intensity, or adding more variety to your workouts. For instance, if you've been focusing on weight lifting, try adding some high-intensity interval training (HIIT) to boost your metabolism and break through plateaus.

Diet adjustments are equally important. Reevaluate your caloric intake and macronutrient distribution. Ensure you're consuming enough protein to support muscle maintenance and repair, and adjust your carbohydrate and fat intake to match your energy needs and goals. Sometimes, a small tweak in your diet can reignite your progress.

Long-Term Maintenance

Achieving your weight loss and muscle maintenance goals is just the beginning. Long-term maintenance involves continuing the healthy habits you've developed. Stay active by incorporating regular physical activity into your daily routine. This doesn't mean you have to stick to the same workout plan indefinitely; feel free to explore different forms of exercise, such as yoga, swimming, or cycling, to keep things interesting and enjoyable.

Healthy eating should remain a priority. Focus on balanced meals that provide the nutrients your body needs to function optimally. Avoid drastic changes in your diet that are unsustainable in the long run. Instead, aim for moderation and consistency.

Staying Motivated

Tracking progress helps you stay motivated by providing tangible proof of your efforts. Celebrate your milestones, no matter how small they may seem. Recognize and reward yourself for the hard work and dedication you've put in. This could be as simple as treating yourself to a new workout outfit, a relaxing massage, or a special meal.

Sharing your journey with others can also boost motivation. Join a fitness community, participate in group workouts, or find a workout buddy. Having a support system can provide encouragement, accountability, and a sense of camaraderie.

In conclusion, tracking your progress is essential for staying motivated and making necessary adjustments to your fitness journey. Regularly measure your body composition, strength gains, and overall fitness. Keep a detailed workout and nutrition journal, adjust your plans as needed, and focus on long-term maintenance. Celebrate your achievements and stay connected with a supportive fitness community. By doing so, you'll stay on track and continue to see progress toward your weight loss and muscle maintenance goals.

Conclusion

Embrace the Comprehensive Approach

Achieving sustainable weight loss and muscle maintenance requires a multifaceted approach. By combining weight lifting with proper nutrition, recovery, and a positive mindset, you lay a solid foundation for long-term success. Each component plays a crucial role:

- **Weight Lifting:** Builds and preserves muscle mass, increases metabolic rate, and contributes to overall strength and functionality.
- **Proper Nutrition:** Fuels your body, supports muscle repair and growth, and helps create a caloric deficit for fat loss.
- **Recovery:** Allows muscles to heal and grow, preventing injuries and enhancing performance.
- **Positive Mindset:** Keeps you motivated, resilient, and focused on your goals, even when challenges arise.

Personalized Journey

Remember, this journey is personal, and everyone's path will be different. Your starting point, progress, and pace will be unique to you. Comparing your journey to others can lead to unnecessary frustration. Instead, focus on your own progress and celebrate your achievements, no matter how small they may seem.

Stay Committed

Consistency is key to any fitness journey. Stay committed to your workout routine, nutrition plan, and recovery practices. There will be times when progress seems slow, or setbacks occur—these are natural parts of the process. What matters is your ability to stay committed and keep moving forward.

Stay Motivated

Find ways to keep yourself motivated. Set short-term and long-term goals, track your progress, and celebrate milestones. Surround yourself with supportive people, whether it's a workout buddy, a fitness community, or an encouraging coach. These connections can provide the encouragement and accountability you need to stay on track.

Enjoy the Process

While the ultimate goal is weight loss and muscle maintenance, it's important to enjoy the process. Find joy in your workouts, savor nutritious meals, and take pride in the progress you make. The journey itself is as important as the destination. By enjoying the process, you're more likely to stay committed and motivated.

A Healthier, Stronger You

At the end of this journey, you won't just be a lighter version of yourself; you'll be healthier, stronger, and more confident. The benefits of this transformation extend beyond the physical. Improved fitness can lead to better mental health, increased energy levels, and a greater sense of accomplishment. You'll find that the discipline and resilience developed in the weight room carry over into other areas of your life.

Glossary of Terms

Afterburn Effect (EPOC)

Excess Post-exercise Oxygen Consumption (EPOC) refers to the increased rate of oxygen intake following strenuous activity intended to erase the body's "oxygen deficit." This effect causes additional calorie burn after exercise as the body returns to its resting state.

Body Composition

The proportion of fat and non-fat mass (muscles, bones, organs, and water) in the body. Improving body composition focuses on reducing fat mass and increasing or maintaining lean mass.

Caloric Deficit

A state where the number of calories consumed is less than the number of calories burned, leading to weight loss. Reducing calorie intake per day by 500 is a good goal.

Cardiovascular Exercise (Cardio)

Physical activity that raises your heart rate and improves the efficiency of the cardiovascular system. Examples include running, swimming, and cycling.

Compound Movements

Exercises that engage multiple muscle groups and joints at the same time. Examples include squats, deadlifts, bench presses, and rows.

Dynamic Stretching

A type of stretching that involves moving parts of your body and gradually increasing reach, speed of movement, or both. It is typically done before workouts to prepare muscles and joints for physical activity.

High-Intensity Interval Training (HIIT)

A cardiovascular exercise strategy alternating short periods of intense anaerobic exercise with less intense recovery periods. HIIT is known for its efficiency in burning calories and improving cardiovascular fitness.

Hydration

The process of ensuring your body has enough fluids to function properly. Proper hydration is essential for maintaining performance, especially during exercise. For longer workouts water should also include carbs and electrolytes.

Isolation Exercises

Exercises that target a specific muscle group using one joint movement. Examples include bicep curls and tricep extensions.

Lean Muscle Mass

The weight of muscle in the body without the fat. It is important for metabolic activity, physical strength, and overall health.

Macronutrients

Nutrients required in large amounts for energy and body functions: proteins, carbohydrates, and fats. Each macronutrient plays a unique role in nutrition and metabolism.

Metabolic Rate

The rate at which your body burns calories to maintain basic physiological functions such as breathing, circulation, and cell production.

Mobility Exercises

Exercises designed to increase the range of motion of joints and improve movement efficiency. They are crucial for maintaining flexibility and preventing injuries.

Periodization

A systematic planning of athletic or physical training. It involves progressive cycling of various aspects of a training program during a specific period.

Progressive Overload

The gradual increase of stress placed upon the body during exercise training. This concept is fundamental for gaining muscle strength and endurance.

Recovery

The process of allowing muscles to repair and grow stronger after exercise. Recovery involves rest, nutrition, hydration, and sleep.

Sarcopenia

The age-related loss of muscle mass and strength. It can significantly affect an individual's physical function and quality of life.

Specificity

The principle that training should be relevant and appropriate to the sport or fitness goal for which the individual is training to produce the desired effect.

Static Stretching

A type of stretching where you hold a single position for a period, allowing muscles to elongate and relax. It is typically done after workouts to aid in recovery.

Testosterone

A hormone that plays a key role in muscle growth, bone mass, and fat distribution. Increased levels can aid in muscle repair and growth.

Weight Lifting (Resistance Training)

A form of exercise that involves lifting weights to build strength and muscle. It includes various types of equipment and techniques, focusing on muscle hypertrophy, strength, and endurance.

ABOUT THE AUTHOR

RUSSELL CAMPBELL
Personal & Group Strength & Conditioning Coach
campbell@yoursecondopinionllc.com
702-816-8430

COACHING & ATHLETIC EXPERIENCE

<u>Sport Conditioning</u>

- Sport Conditioning Fitness Classes at D1 Training, Sun City Aliante. Summerlin Reverence in Las Vegas NV: Golf, Tennis & Pickleball Athletes – Strength, Power & Injury Prevention
- Personal strength & power training with individual senior golf, pickleballers and tennis players

<u>Weightlifting</u>

- Provincial Senior Champion – 3x, Multiple time Canadian Masters Champion, PanAm Masters Champion. World Masters Silver Medalist
- Coached by Steve Sandor for 6 years, former Hungarian professional weightlifter; he trained 11 athletes who competed in the Olympics, PanAm & Commonwealth Games
- Trained for 6 years with Akos Sandor – Olympian, Silver medalist at World Juniors

- Have trained with many national level athletes & international team members. Briefly trained with Antonio Krastev, former superheavyweight record-holder in Snatch

<u>Other Power Sports</u>
- College football – Conference All – Star; Phi Delta Theta Fraternity All – American , 11 years of amateur football - played with and against many D1 collegiate players and future pros
- Highland Games – Previously ranked in top 15 in age category, Have attended throwing clinics with top-ranked coaches and athletes, Trained with collegiate coaches for shot put, discus, hammer, Advised recent Highland Games World Champion on programming
- Powerlifting – Past provincial record holder
- High school & club athlete – Basketball, football, wrestling, track & field, volleyball, badminton, hockey, baseball, judo

EDUCATION AND PROFESSIONAL DESIGNATIONS

- **Certified Strength & Conditioning Specialist (CSCS), NSCA-** applied scientific knowledge to train athletes for the primary goal of improving athletic performance. Conduct sport-specific testing sessions, design and implement safe and effective strength training and conditioning programs and provide guidance regarding nutrition and injury prevention
- **Olympic Weightlifting Coach - Level 2 (advanced), USAW-** scientifically based program design, technique, lift progressions, assessing movement, motor learning, biomechanics, effective coaching, error correction

- AMP, Advanced Management Program. INSEAD, Paris, France
- MBA, Finance & Marketing, York University, Toronto, Canada
- BA, Industrial Relations, McGill University, Montreal, Canada
- Chartered Financial Analyst, Certified Financial Planner